SICKLE CELL DISEASE
A guide for families

by

Elizabeth N Anionwu and Harun B Jibril

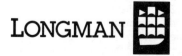

Acknowledgements

The Authors and Publishers are grateful to the following for permission to reproduce copyright material in this guide.

This edition has been adapted from the original handbook written by Elizabeth Anionwu and June Hall and published by the Sickle Cell Society of Great Britain in 1983.

Illustrations by Anthea Eames.

Design, maps and diagrams by Wendi Watson.
The diagrams on pp 13, 29, 69 are adapted from original illustrations by Bryan Jones.

Malaria map on p 35 reproduced by permission of Sutton-Siebert Publications.

The salt-sugar solution drawing on p 34 reproduced by permission of the Tropical Child Health Unit of the Institute of Child Health, University of London.

Cover photo by permission of Ade Onibokun.

First published 1986
Fourth impression 1995

ISBN 0 582 09138 1

Phototypeset by Input Typesetting Ltd, London
Produced through Longman Malaysia, ETS

Published by **Longman Group Limited**
Longman House, Burnt Mill, Harlow,
Essex CM20 2JE, England
and Associated Companies
throughout the world

Sickle cell disease: a guide for families

Sickle cell disease is the name of a group of inherited disorders of haemoglobin. There are several different kinds of sickle cell disease but these three are the most common:

1 Sickle cell anaemia (Hb SS) This is the most well known. It is found in about 1 out of every 200 babies of West African origin and about 1 in 300 babies of Afro-Caribbean origin. It occurs when a child inherits sickle haemoglobin (Hb S) from both parents.

2 SC disease (Hb SC) This is generally less common at birth except in Ghana, and is usually less serious. It occurs when a child inherits sickle haemoglobin (Hb S) from one parent and haemoglobin C (Hb C) from the other.

3 Sickle beta-thalassaemia (Hb S Beta-thal) This occurs when a child inherits sickle haemoglobin (Hb S) from one parent and beta-thalassaemia (Beta-thal) from the other.

This guide gives more details about these three kinds of sickle cell disease, why they happen, and how to look after somebody who has sickle cell disease.

List of Contents

We have divided this book into sections to make it easier to use. However, you don't have to read it straight through from beginning to end. You may prefer to turn straight to the sections that interest you.

(1) Introduction

We have written this guide mainly for families affected by sickle cell disease. We hope that it will help you understand more about what sickle cell disease is, how it is inherited, and how to cope with any problems and difficulties that you may run into.

We have based the guide on our own experiences with families affected by sickle cell disease, and we have tried to answer the questions that people most often ask us. We have also tried to use simple language, and to avoid complicated medical terms. (The glossary in section **14** gives simple explanations of the medical words we have had to use).

You will notice that we have used 'may', 'perhaps' and 'sometimes' a lot in this guide. This is for two reasons. Firstly, we do not want to be too definite. Not everyone with sickle cell disease has the same symptoms or problems. Every person is different. Secondly, doctors and nurses may not always give the same advice. Doctors in different areas may have different ideas and ways of treating sickle cell disease. Research is also producing new ideas and some doctors are more up-to-date than others.

If you are reading this guide because you, or someone you know, has sickle cell disease, you may first want to know exactly what kind of sickle cell disease it is. We suggest that you ask your doctor. If you have any difficulties please contact the most convenient address listed in section **12**.

We should like to thank all the people who helped in the preparation of the original handbook, especially June Hall, and those who have advised us in this guide, with special thanks to Dr. Milica Brozovic, Professor Graham Serjeant and Professor Huxley Knox-Macaulay.

We hope that families throughout the world will find the information useful.

Elizabeth N. Anionwu and Harun B. Jibril

May 1985

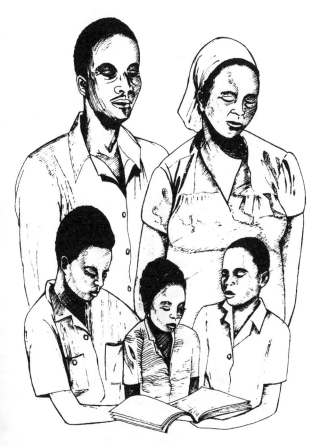

② What is sickle cell disease?

We have found that people are often confused and disturbed by some of the incorrect information they have received about sickle cell disease. So we will start by reassuring you about some of the **wrong** things you may have heard.

SICKLE CELL DISEASE
- IS **NOT** LEUKAEMIA
- IS **NOT** CANCER
- IS **NOT** WHITE BLOOD CELLS EATING UP RED BLOOD CELLS
- IS **NOT** INFECTIOUS — YOU CAN'T 'CATCH IT' LIKE YOU CAN 'CATCH' MEASLES OR A COLD

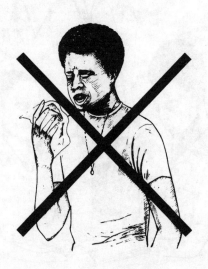

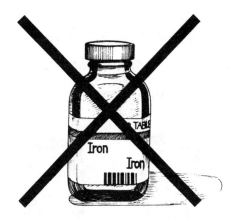

Obviously there is much more to know about what sickle cell disease is. We will start off here with just a few very important things. We discuss them all in more detail further on.

SICKLE CELL DISEASE
   IS INHERITED FROM **BOTH** PARENTS

SICKLE CELL TRAIT

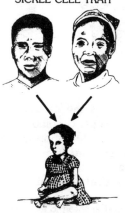

SICKLE CELL ANAEMIA

IS A CONDITION WHICH AFFECTS THE **BLOOD**

IS CAUSED BY A SPECIAL KIND OF **HAEMO-GLOBIN** IN THE RED BLOOD CELLS

IS A DISEASE THAT **MAINLY** AFFECTS PEOPLE OF AFRO-CARIBBEAN* ORIGIN, **BUT ALSO** PEOPLE OF MEDITERRANEAN, ASIAN AND ARAB ORIGIN (see the map on page 22)

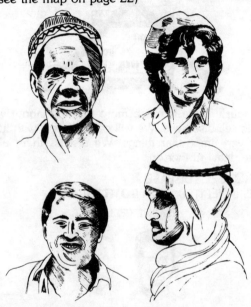

Sickle cell disease is the medical name for several similar but **different** conditions. The three most common kinds of sickle cell disease are:

Sickle cell anaemia
SC disease
Sickle Beta-thalassaemia

---

* We have used Afro-Caribbean to mean people from Africa and people of African origin from the West Indies.

③ How does sickle cell disease affect the blood?

Sickle cell disease affects the haemoglobin in the red blood cells. It sometimes makes the red blood cells change their shape, and this can cause pain and other problems.

3.1 What do red blood cells do?

Blood is made up of several different parts. Each does a different job. The following make up the four main parts.

Plasma is the liquid part of blood which carries all the other parts round the body to where they are needed.

Red blood cells make blood look red and are normally round. They carry oxygen from the lungs all round the body in a substance called **haemoglobin.** Sickle cell disease affects the haemoglobin in the red blood cells.

White blood cells help to destroy bacteria and to heal cuts and injuries.

Platelets help the blood to clot if people cut themselves.

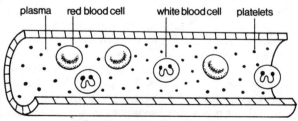

Section through a blood vessel

11

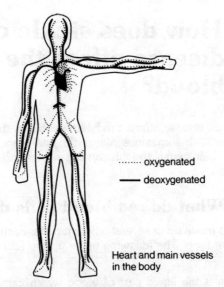

oxygenated
deoxygenated

Heart and main vessels
in the body

3.2 What does haemoglobin do?

Haemoglobin is a substance in the red blood cells that carries oxygen. The red blood cells pick up the oxygen in the lungs and travel with it round the body. They release the oxygen wherever it is needed.

3.3 Are there different kinds of haemoglobin?

Yes, there are about 300 different kinds. The most common kind is haemoglobin A. (A stands for adult). The kinds which are most important in sickle cell disease are sickle haemoglobin and haemoglobin C. Thalassaemia, a condition in which the body cannot make enough haemoglobin, is also important.

The kind of haemoglobin anybody has depends on what they inherited from their parents. Most people inherit haemoglobin A. Some people inherit other kinds. (To find out more about inheritance, see section **4**.)

3.4 What does sickle haemoglobin do?

When red blood cells with ordinary haemoglobin (haemoglobin A) release oxygen they remain round. But a person who has sickle cell disease has mainly sickle haemoglobin in their red blood cells. When red blood cells with sickle haemoglobin release oxygen, they sometimes change shape. They then look like a farmer's sickle or a crescent moon. This is where the name 'sickle' cell comes from.

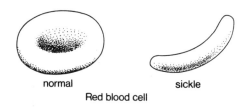

normal   sickle

Red blood cell

These sickle cells cannot flow through the very narrow blood vessels in the body. This is called sickling. They often get stuck and stop the blood flowing and it can cause a **painful crisis**.

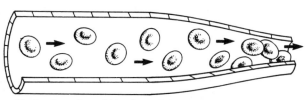

Section through small blood vessel showing normal flow of blood

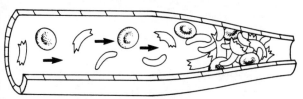

Section through small blood vessel showing sickling

13

During a crisis the sickled blood cells can cause a lot of pain. They sometimes form a clot and can damage parts of the body. In section **5** we tell you how to try and prevent somebody with sickle cell disease having a sickle crisis and what to do if they have one.

4 How do people get sickle cell disease?

Sickle cell disease is **inherited**. This means that people are born with it, just as they are born with other characteristics such as eye colour, hair texture and height. It is inherited from **both** parents.

If you are not born with sickle cell disease you will never get it, because it is **not** infectious. You **cannot** catch it.

4.1 How does inheritance work?

Let's start at the beginning. A child comes into being when the father's sperm joins with the egg of the mother.

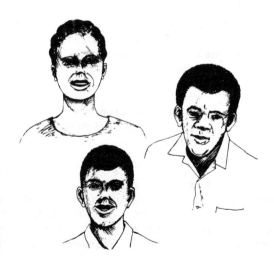

When the child is born nine months later people may notice that it resembles both its parents in different ways. For example, our illustration on p 15 shows that the child has inherited his father's ears and hairline and his mother's round face and pointed nose. These resemblances are called characteristics. They are passed on from parents to children by substances called genes, in the father's sperm and the mother's egg. There are thousands of different genes in the sperm and the egg, all for different characteristics, and all passed on to the child. For example, there are genes for height, eye colour, hair texture, foot size and so on, and also for haemoglobin. So you inherit the kind of haemoglobin you have in your red blood cells from both your mother and your father.

4.2 What kind of haemoglobin did I inherit?

Everybody inherits two genes, one from each parent. These are the most important genes involved in sickle cell disease and trait:

The most common gene is **haemoglobin A**
(often written as **Hb*A**)
Then there are **sickle haemoglobin**
(often written as **Hb S**)
and **haemoglobin C**
(often written as **Hb C**)
and **beta-thalassaemia**
(often written as **Beta-thal** or
B-thal)

*Hb is the short form for haemoglobin.

If you inherited, for example, two genes for haemoglobin A (Hb A) you will have haemoglobin AA (Hb AA), normal haemoglobin. If you inherited one gene for haemoglobin A (Hb A) and one for sickle haemoglobin (Hb S), you will have sickle cell trait (Hb

16

AS). Sickle cell trait is not a disease. (see section **4.4**).

Do you know what kind of haemoglobin you inherited? You can easily have a test to find out. Section **8.1** tells you how to get the test.

Here are the most common kinds of haemoglobin. You have probably inherited one of these:

HAEMOGLOBIN TYPE	USUALLY CALLED	
Hb AA	**normal haemoglobin**	
Hb AS	**sickle cell trait**	⎫
Hb AC	**C trait**	⎬ **traits**
Hb A Beta-thal	**thalassaemia trait**	⎭
HB SS	**sickle cell anaemia**	⎫ **kinds of**
Hb SC	**SC disease**	⎬ **sickle cell**
Hb S Beta-thal	**sickle beta-thalassaemia**	⎭ **disease**

4.3 How do people inherit normal haemoglobin?

HAEMOGLOBIN AA
normal haemoglobin

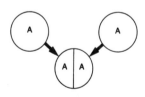

If you have haemoglobin AA (Hb AA) you inherited haemoglobin A (Hb A) from both your parents. Haemoglobin AA is what most people have. It causes no problems. (Doctors and other people often shorten haemoglobin AA to haemoglobin A. It means the same and you may hear both).

4.4 How do people inherit sickle cell trait?

HAEMOGLOBIN AS
Sickle cell trait

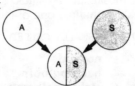

If you have sickle cell trait (Hb AS), you inherited haemoglobin A (Hb A) from one parent, and sickle haemoglobin (Hb S) from the other. You have mainly haemoglobin A.

The word 'trait' means that you do not have the disease but that you could possibly pass it on to your children. People with a trait are often said to be 'carriers'; they do not have it themselves, but they carry the gene and could pass it on to their children.

(In very, very unusual circumstances people with sickle cell trait may get some blood in their urine, because they have sickling in their kidneys. They do not become ill).

There are other kinds of trait; the main ones are:

HAEMOGLOBIN AC
C trait

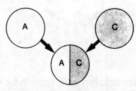

If you have C trait (Hb AC), you inherited haemoglobin A (Hb A) from one parent and haemoglobin C (Hb C) from the other. You have mainly haemoglobin A. Haemoglobin C does not cause problems by itself, but it can when combined with other unusual haemoglobins. People with C trait have no health problems though they carry haemoglobin C and could pass it on to their children.

HAEMOGLOBIN A BETA-THAL
Thalassaemia trait

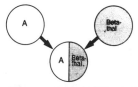

If you have thalassaemia trait (Hb A Beta-thal), you inherited haemoglobin A (Hb A) from one parent and beta-thalassaemia (Beta-thal) from the other. You have mainly haemoglobin A. People with thalassaemia trait are healthy but they carry the thalassaemia gene and could pass it on to their children. (For more about thalassaemia see section **7**.)

If you have a trait, for example, sickle cell trait, C trait or thalassaemia trait
It is **not** an illness
It is **not** infectious
It will **not** make you feel ill
It will **not** change to sickle cell disease
You inherited it from your parents and were **born** with it
But if **both** you and your partner have a trait your children **could** inherit sickle cell disease.
You have the trait because you inherited a gene for the usual haemoglobin, haemoglobin A, from one parent, and a gene for a different haemoglobin from your other parent. You have mainly haemoglobin A, so you do not get the problems of sickle cell disease.

4.5 How do people inherit sickle cell disease?

HAEMOGLOBIN SS
Sickle cell anaemia

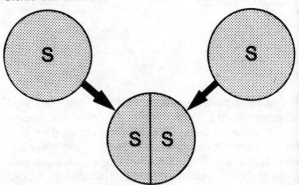

If you have sickle cell anaemia you inherited one sickle cell gene (Hb S) from each of your parents. This is the most common kind of sickle cell disease. (To find out more about sickle cell anaemia, the problems it may cause and how to manage them, see section **5**).

HAEMOGLOBIN SC
SC disease

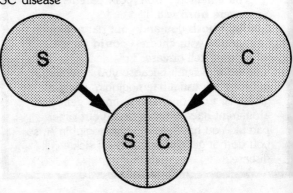

If you have SC disease (Hb SC), you inherited a sickle cell gene (Hb S) from one parent and a haemoglobin C gene (Hb C) from the other. (Please note that SC disease is **not** the same as sickle cell anaemia and is a kind of sickle cell disease.)

Haemoglobin C by itself does not cause problems, but when it is combined with sickle haemoglobin it may cause red blood cells to sickle. SC disease is usually not as serious as sickle cell anaemia. (We say more about SC disease in section **6**.)

HAEMOGLOBIN S BETA-THAL
Sickle Beta-thalassaemia

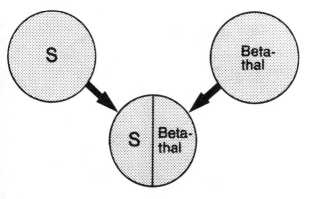

If you have sickle beta-thalassaemia (Hb S Beta-thal) you inherited a sickle cell gene (Hb S) from one parent and a beta-thalassaemia gene (Beta-thal) from the other. People with sickle beta-thalassaemia sometimes get sickling of red blood cells. (We say more about sickle beta-thalassaemia in section **7**.)

There are also other kinds of sickle cell disease such as S with hereditary persistence of fetal haemoglobin (S/HPFH), SD Punjab, and SO Arab disease. If you would like more information please contact the nearest society/centre listed on p 83.

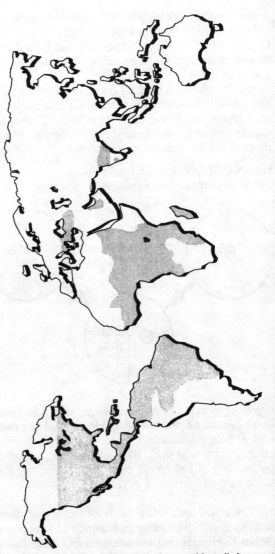

Map of the world showing areas where sickle cell disease is found.

22

- The different kinds of sickle cell disease and the different traits, are found mainly in people whose families come from Africa, the West Indies, the Middle East, the Eastern Mediterranean, and Asia (see the map on page 22.)
- This is because sickle cell trait, (and possibly C trait and thalassaemia trait) can protect children from malaria, a serious disease which often kills children in these parts of the world. (see section **5.4** on malaria.)
- Sickle cell trait is found in about 1 out of every 10 people (10%) of Afro-Caribbean origin (and more frequently in Nigeria).
- C trait is found in about 1 out of every 50 people (2%) of Afro-Caribbean origin and about 1 in 5 (20%) in Ghana.
- Thalassaemia trait is found in about 1 out of every 50 people (2%) of Afro-Caribbean origin (and more frequently in Mediterranean countries).

4.6 What about my children? What will they inherit?

Your children will inherit one haemoglobin gene from you and one from your partner. You will remember that you inherited two genes from your parents and that your partner also inherited two genes. Which two out of these four genes will each of your children inherit?

That is a matter of chance. Each child will inherit **one** of your two genes and **one** of your partner's two genes. Nobody can foretell which genes the child will inherit. So you cannot tell in advance exactly what kind of haemoglobin your child will have. However, if you know what kinds of haemoglobin you and your partner have, **you know the possibilities**.

What are the possibilities? Let us look at some examples.

Take 4 couples:

Couple One   In this couple, the woman has normal haemoglobin (Hb AA) and the man has sickle cell trait (Hb AS).

This means that the woman has two genes for haemoglobin A, and the man has one gene for haemoglobin A and one for sickle haemoglobin.

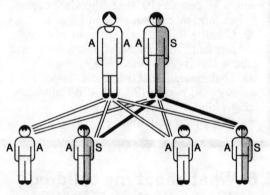

If they have a child, it may inherit haemoglobin A from both parents, in which case it will have normal haemoglobin (Hb AA);
or it may inherit normal haemoglobin (Hb A) from its mother, and sickle haemoglobin (Hb S) from its father, in which case it will have sickle cell trait (Hb AS).

You can see from the diagram above that out of the four possibilities, two are for normal haemoglobin (Hb AA) and two are for sickle cell trait (Hb AS). **For each child** this couple has there is a 1 in 2 (50%)

24

chance it will have normal haemoglobin (Hb AA) and a 1 in 2 (50%) chance that it will have sickle cell trait (Hb AS).

Couple Two In this couple, both parents have sickle cell trait (Hb AS). So each parent has one gene for sickle haemoglobin and one for haemoglobin A, normal haemoglobin.

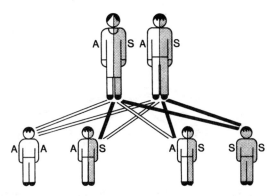

If they have a child it may inherit haemoglobin A from both parents, in which case it will have normal haemoglobin, haemoglobin AA (Hb AA);
or it may inherit sickle haemoglobin from both parents, in which case it will have sickle cell anaemia (Hb SS);
or it may inherit sickle haemoglobin from one parent and normal haemoglobin, haemoglobin A (Hb A), from the other, in which case it will have sickle cell trait (Hb AS).

Out of the four possibilities, two are for sickle cell trait (Hb AS), one is for sickle cell anaemia (Hb SS) and one is for normal haemoglobin (Hb AA). So **for each child** this couple has, there is a 1 in 2 (50%) chance it will have sickle cell trait; a 1 in 4 (25%) chance it will have sickle cell anaemia, and a 1 in 4 (25%) chance it will have normal haemoglobin.

Couple Three In this couple, the woman has sickle cell anaemia (Hb SS) and the man has sickle cell trait (Hb AS).

This means that the woman has two genes for sickle haemoglobin, and the man has one gene for sickle haemoglobin and one for normal haemoglobin, haemoglobin A.

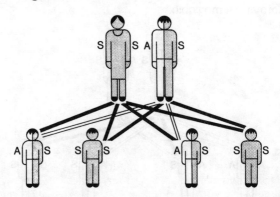

If they have a child it may inherit sickle haemoglobin from both parents, in which case it will have sickle cell anaemia (Hb SS);
or it may inherit sickle haemoglobin from its mother, and normal haemoglobin, haemoglobin A, from its father, in which case it will have sickle cell trait (Hb AS).

Out of the four possibilities, two are for sickle cell anaemia (Hb SS) and two are for sickle cell trait (Hb AS). So, **for each child** this couple has there is a 1 in 2 (50%) chance that it will have sickle cell anaemia and a 1 in 2 (50%) chance that it will have sickle cell trait.

Couple Four In this couple, the woman has sickle cell trait (Hb AS), and the man has C trait (Hb AC).

This means that the woman has one gene for normal haemoglobin and one gene for sickle haemoglobin. The man has one gene for normal haemoglobin and one gene for haemoglobin C.

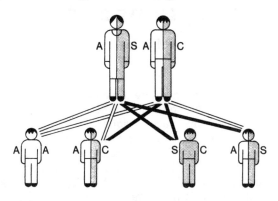

If they have a child it may inherit normal haemoglobin from both parents, in which case it will have normal haemoglobin, haemoglobin AA (Hb AA);
or it may inherit normal haemoglobin from its mother and haemoglobin C from its father, in which case it will have C trait (Hb AC);
or it may inherit sickle haemoglobin from its mother and haemoglobin C from its father, in which case it will have SC disease (Hb SC);
or it may inherit sickle haemoglobin from its mother and normal haemoglobin from its father, in which case it will have sickle cell trait (Hb AS).

Out of the four possibilities, one is for normal haemoglobin (Hb AA), one is for C trait (Hb AC), one is for SC disease (Hb SC) and one is for sickle cell trait (Hb AS). So **for each child** this couple has there is a 1 in 4 (25%) chance that it will have normal haemoglobin; a 1 in 4 (25%) chance that it will have C trait; a 1 in 4 (25%) chance that it will have SC disease; and a 1 in 4 (25%) chance that it will have sickle cell trait.

⑤ Sickle cell anaemia (Hb SS): symptoms and problems

As we have said, there are three main kinds of sickle cell disease: sickle cell anaemia, SC disease, and sickle beta-thalassaemia. Each is slightly different.

The most common kind of sickle cell disease among people of Afro-Caribbean origin is sickle cell anaemia, so we will describe this first and most fully. In sections **6** and **7** we describe SC disease and sickle beta-thalassaemia much more briefly and outline the differences between them and sickle cell anaemia. **Whatever kind of sickle cell disease you are interested in, please read the whole of section 5 first as much of it also applies to SC disease and sickle beta-thalassaemia**.

At present there is no cure for sickle cell disease. So a person born with any kind of sickle cell disease has it for life. However, some of the problems that people with sickle cell disease get can be treated and some of them can be prevented. In section **9** we give a list of hints which people with sickle cell disease have found useful in helping them to live a reasonably normal life.

5.1 Sickle cell anaemia (Hb SS)

Sickle cell anaemia occurs when a child inherits sickle haemoglobin (Hb S) from both parents. Sickle cell anaemia is found in 1 in 500 babies in the USA, about one in every 300 babies of Afro-Caribbean origin and 1 in every 100 babies in many African communities.

Sickle cell anaemia affects the haemoglobin in the red blood cells. Sickle haemoglobin can sometimes cause a person's red blood cells to become sickle shaped (see section **3**). This is called 'sickling'. They then become stuck in the small blood vessels blocking the flow of blood in the body.

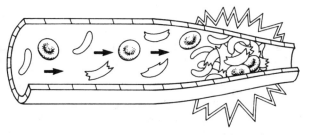

5.2 What causes sickling?

HERE ARE SOME OF THE MAIN CAUSES:

1 Reduced supply of oxygen to various parts of the body. For example, this can be caused by **strenuous exercise**. Normal exercise is all right. Too much may cause sickling. Each person knows how much they can take.

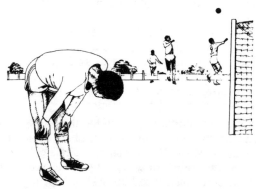

2 Anaesthetics Gases or drugs used before an operation to put people to sleep. Anaesthetics can be more dangerous for people with sickle cell disease because they may cause sickling through lack of oxygen and dehydration. If doctors know you have the disease they can take care to prevent sickling. If you are going to have an anaesthetic you **must** tell doctors, dentists or nurses that you have sickle cell disease.

3 Dehydration Too little liquid in the body. This can happen if a person has not drunk enough; if they have been very hot or have perspired after exercise; or because of diarrhoea or vomiting. (see section **5.3**.)

4 Infection For example, malaria (see section **5.4**), a chest infection or pneumonia.

5 Fever A high temperature.

6 Pregnancy This is because of some of the changes a woman's body goes through when she is pregnant. Pregnancy increases the risk that the red blood cells will sickle though nobody yet really understands all the reasons. However, malaria is known to cause sickling in pregnancy (see section **5.4**). Doctors and nurses will want to keep a careful check on any woman who is pregnant to make sure she is all right. If you have sickle cell disease tell your doctor or medical adviser as soon as you know you are pregnant. (See the section on pregnancy in **5.9**.)

7 Sudden changes in temperature For example, going from a warm room into a cold place.

8 Alcohol Alcohol may lead to sickling by causing dehydration.

9 Emotional stress For example, feeling under pressure, exam stress, depression.

It is very important to know the things that cause sickling so that you can be careful to avoid them as far as possible. But sometimes sickling happens **without anybody knowing why**. One of the most common problems caused by sickling is pain.

5.3 Dehydration

WHAT IS DEHYDRATION?

Dehydration is a condition which occurs when water is lost from the body and is not adequately replaced.

Water is very important to our body, in fact over two thirds of our body is made up of water; it is in our cells and is an essential part of our blood and other body fluids. Therefore lack of water, (dehydration), makes our body cells 'dry', just as a fresh pea seed dries by wrinkling and shrivelling when left to dry.

In persons who have sickle cell disease dehydration causes the blood to thicken; this disturbs the normal smooth flow in the blood vessels; it becomes sluggish and therefore causes the red blood cells to sickle. Thus a crisis results. It is most important to keep the blood thin and flowing, so **a person suffering from sickle cell disease must drink a lot of water in order to avoid a crisis**.

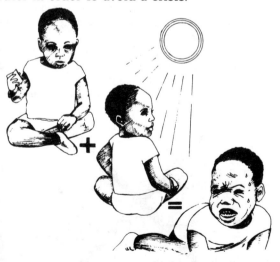

SICKLE CELL DISEASE + DEHYDRATION = SICKLE CELL CRISIS

WHAT CAUSES DEHYDRATION?

In Africa, and indeed most tropical areas of the world, temperatures in the environment are high; people are therefore constantly losing water through their skin by sweating and also through their breathing. Persons with sickle cell disease living in these areas must keep drinking almost all the time to prevent getting dehydrated.

Another major cause of dehydration in the tropics is **gastroenteritis**. This is a condition in which there is diarrhoea and vomiting which causes water and salts to be lost from the intestines.

There are many causes of gastroenteritis:

1 **Infections** in the gut with bacteria (such as cholera and dysentry) and viruses are common causes of diarrhoea and vomiting. Infections elsewhere in the body can also cause diarrhoea and vomiting; for example malaria, chest and ear infections. In addition, these infections are usually associated with high fever, which causes sweating, and this makes the dehydration worse.
2 **Poisons** that are harmful to the intestines, for example, those produced by bacteria in cooked food that is then left overnight.
3 **Use of dirty bottles and cups** for feeding children.

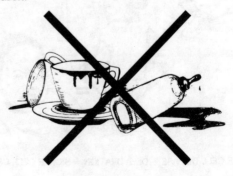

4 Too much pepper in food. Meals prepared with a lot of pepper irritate the intestine, and can cause diarrhoea.

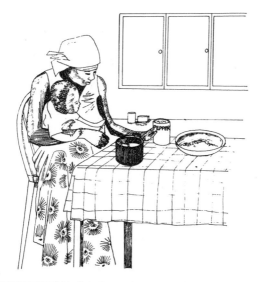

PREVENTION OF DEHYDRATION

1 Drinking plenty of water is the most important preventive measure.

2 Try to avoid excessive exercise or too much exertion; this leads to loss of water and so results in dehydration.

3 Keep immediate surroundings clean. This will prevent food becoming infected.

4 Always use clean utensils in food preparation, especially when feeding children. They are most easily affected by dehydration if they have diarrhoea or vomiting.

TREATMENT OF DEHYDRATION

● Mild dehydration can be treated at home with simple rehydration (replacement) fluid that can be easily prepared: **the salt-sugar solution**. The correct mixture is obtained by dissolving 'thumb and two fingers pinch' of salt and 'four finger scoop' of sugar in a mug of water.

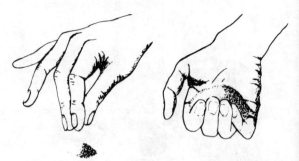

Thumb + 2 fingers pinch   The four finger scoop of sugar = 30g

Salt - sugar rehydration solution

This treatment is especially suitable for children.
The child is given as much of the solution as he can tolerate until dehydration is corrected.
● Currently there are rehydration powders available, prepared by the World Health Organisation. These can be dissolved and given to dehydrated persons.
● Moderate to severe dehydration is best treated in the health centre or hospital. So if dehydration is not corrected by drinking a lot of water or salt-sugar solution **do not delay seeking help in the hospital**.
● If there is any underlying cause of the dehydration, this must be treated adequately, to avoid sickle crisis.

5.4 Malaria

Malaria is still common in many areas of the world such as Africa, India, South East Asia, Central and South America. Sickle cell disease is also common in these areas. Sickle cell trait offers some protection

34

against malaria but sickle cell disease **does not**; malaria can be fatal in a person with sickle cell disease. In this section we shall be discussing the affects of malaria on sickle cell disease as well as signs, symptoms, prevention and treatment of malaria.

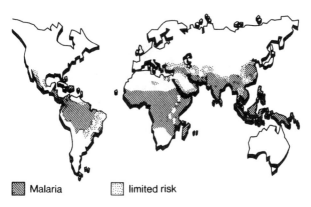

▨ Malaria   ▦ limited risk

Map of the world showing distribution of malaria

WHAT IS MALARIA?

Malaria is an infection caused by a small parasite called *Plasmodium*. It is spread by mosquitoes. There are four important types of *Plasmodium: Falciparum* (the commonest in Africa), *Malariae, Ovale*, and *Vivax*. (see above map).

In West Africa the female *Anopheles* mosquito is the important carrier. This is because it feeds on human blood before it is able to lay its eggs. Therefore, if the mosquito feeds on a person that has the malarial parasite in his blood, it carries the parasite and injects it into the next person it bites.

The mosquito breeds on stagnant water, usually around houses, such as in gutters, empty containers left to collect rain water and in shrubs surrounding the compound.

35

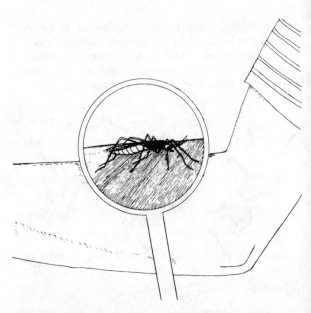

HOW DOES MALARIA AFFECT THE BLOOD?

When the mosquito bites a person, it injects the parasite into the bloodstream. After passing through the liver, it then enters into the circulation where it uses up oxygen, multiplies, and destroys the red blood cells. This process is constantly repeated and this is why a person can have repeated attacks of malaria.

WHAT ARE THE SYMPTOMS?

The main symptom is fever which usually starts about 10 to 15 days after a mosquito bite. It begins with shivering and tiredness, and ends with intense sweating, following which the person will feel some relief before the next attack sets in. Other symptoms include headache, nausea and vomiting and stomach upset. Diarrhoea and vomiting are more common in children, as a result of which they can become easily dehydrated (see page 44). The spleen and the liver enlarge in a few days. Malaria can also cause the following severe complications: convulsions (fits), cerebral malaria (malaria in the brain), severe anaemia, kidney problems and swelling of the body.

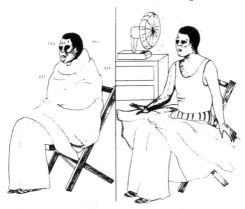

TREATMENT OF MALARIA

Prompt treatment is necessary to prevent the serious complications of malaria, especially in a person with sickle cell disease. **As soon as you notice any symptom of malaria, visit your nearest hospital or health centre so that appropriate treatment may be given.**

Several drugs can be used to treat malaria. It is important to contact a doctor or local health officer so that correct doses of these drugs are given and treatment is properly carried out.

THINGS TO REMEMBER ABOUT TREATMENT OF MALARIA

1 Preventive tablets must be taken regularly to ensure good protection. When you miss a dose, contact your health centre for advice.

2 Avoid 'shot-gun' treatment. Do not buy medicines from road-side stores without medical advice; you are more likely to buy the wrong medicine and take the wrong dosage, therefore causing malarial parasites to become resistant to medicine.

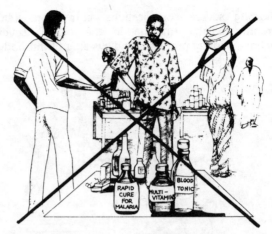

3 When complications occur (see p 36), do not delay going to the hospital for treatment.
4 Remember that all medicine is potential poison, so keep it out of reach of children.

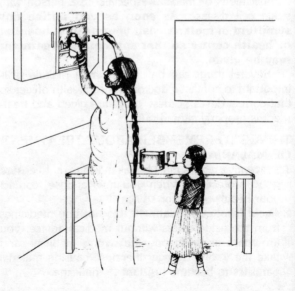

MALARIA AND SICKLE CELL TRAIT

Children under the age of five years, who have sickle cell trait, have some protection against malaria. They are therefore much less affected. This partly explains why sickle cell trait is frequently found in areas where malaria is common. This, however, is **not** the case for children with sickle cell disease who do not have such protection. In fact malaria in sickle cell disease is a very serious problem and can lead to sudden death, as will be explained later. **It is therefore most important to prevent malaria in every person with sickle cell disease.**

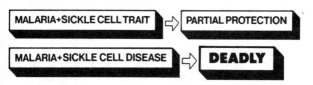

MALARIA AND SICKLE CELL DISEASE

As mentioned earlier, malarial parasites affect the red blood cells. When the parasite infects a person with sickle cell disease, they enter the red blood cells, use up the oxygen carried in them and cause them to sickle. This occurs very quickly and affects a large number of the red blood cells; it therefore results in a severe sickle crisis. **Malaria is a very common cause of sickle crisis in tropical areas**.

SICKLE CELL DISEASE, PREGNANCY AND MALARIA

Pregnant women usually have reduced resistance to infections, including malarial infection. Pregnant women with sickle cell disease are therefore very prone to having attacks of malaria. Their red blood cells are destroyed at a much faster rate, so that they do not only get severe crises, but also severe anaemia. They have an increased need for **folic acid** too, which, if not taken, makes the anaemia worse. If they are not treated, abortion of the foetus or premature labour leading to the delivery of the baby too early and possibly too small to survive results. These are in addition to the affects of malaria on the mother.

It is therefore **essential** that pregnant women with sickle cell disease take **malaria preventive tablets** as well as folic acid regularly. **They should go to the hospital or the nearest health centre for advice if they develop any symptoms of malaria.**

HOW CAN MALARIA BE PREVENTED?

It is vital that individuals with sickle cell disease be protected against malaria. This can be achieved in a variety of ways:

1 The Household

  a) Try to keep your compounds clean. Do not leave empty containers in the surroundings, these will provide breeding places for the mosquito.

  b) Clear away thick shrubs and drain any water collection in and around the house. If there are areas with collections of water that cannot be drained, they can be sprayed with substances that make the water surface unsuitable for the larval stages of the mosquitoes to survive. In some areas of the world, certain fishes that feed on these larval worms control mosquito breeding.

  c) If wells are used as a source of water build some concrete parapets around them and provide covers for them.

  d) Provide wire netting for all windows and doors in the house. Windows should be large enough to allow for adequate illumination in the rooms, as mosquitoes tend to hide in dark areas.

  e) Rooms can be sprayed with insecticides that kill adult mosquitoes. This is commonly done in urban areas where such insecticides are available.

2) Man

  a) Always wear protective clothing to bed.

  b) Use mosquito nets to prevent mosquitoes from

40

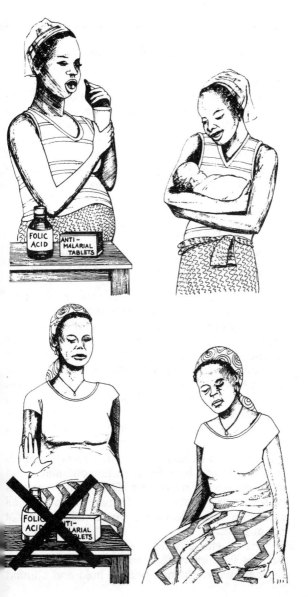

coming into contact with exposed parts of the body when retiring.

c) creams are available for applying on the body; they stop mosquitoes from biting us.

3) Medicine

This is an important preventive measure. For it to succeed, **the medicine must be taken regularly**. If you are on a regular antimalarial preventive drug, and you forget to take a dose, contact your hospital or health centre for advice on how to make up for the missed dose. Protection cannot be guaranteed once a dose is missed.

5.5 What should I do if somebody has a painful crisis because of sickling?

1 Encourage them to tell you as soon as the pain makes them feel very uncomfortable.

2 Make them comfortable on a bed or a couch.

3 Encourage them to drink plenty of liquids, for example, water, squash, milk or fruit juice (but **not** fizzy drinks as these might make the stomach more uncomfortable). Someone with a painful crisis should drink at least one glass of liquid every hour. This will thin the blood and help stop the sickling. Put a full jug and a glass beside them. Keep filling the jug.

4 Give the pain killers the doctor has recommended. Allow up to one hour for them to work. Make sure there are always some pain killers in the house as pain can start at any time. Remember to keep all medicines in a locked place where children cannot get at them.

5 A person who is having a sickle cell crisis may become very frightened and tense. This can make the pain worse. It may help to hold and comfort

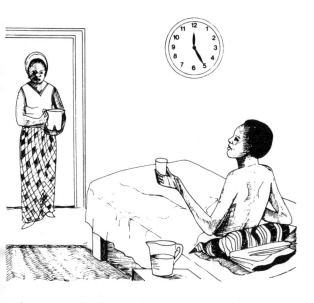

them to make them relax and feel safe. Encourage them to talk about their feelings and fear.

If you do all this as soon as someone becomes unwell, the pains usually begin to go away.

5.6 When should I seek medical help?

IF THE PAIN GOES ON GETTING WORSE, OR DOES NOT GO AWAY **SEEK MEDICAL HELP IMMEDIATELY.**
Take the person to the nearest hospital or health centre if someone with a sickle cell crisis shows any one of the following symptoms:

● has a high temperature (over 38.0°C or 100.4°F)
● has severe pain anywhere in their body, especially if the pain goes on after the person has taken pain killers, but remember to allow up to one hour for the

43

pain killers to start working. (If you are unhappy about the pain killers you have at home discuss this with your doctor).

● has a cough that will not go away
● has a bad headache, seems very sleepy and/or weakness down one side of the body
● has diarrhoea or vomiting, or cannot keep down liquids
● is short of breath, cannot breathe properly
● is listless, has no energy
● suddenly becomes pale
● gets very yellow eyes
● has a painful erection or pain in the private parts (penis), at any time.

If you are looking after a young child with a painful crisis, it is most important to take them to hospital if they suddenly get a bad tummy pain or a swollen and tender tummy. This could mean that red blood cells are sickling in the spleen (see the section on splenic sequestration in **5.8**) **This needs urgent attention.**

5.7 What other problems might people with sickle cell disease have?

It is important to remember that the effects of sickle cell disease vary a lot from person to person. Most people have long periods when they feel fine, known as the 'steady state', and sometimes, periods when they feel ill.

Below, we have made a list of all the **possible** problems that people with sickle cell anaemia and other sickle cell diseases **may** have. But please note that most people have only a few of these. We have listed them all here because many people have told us that they would prefer to know about things **before** they happen.

In section **5.8** we describe the symptoms and

problems a young child might have. In section **5.9** we describe problems that can affect teenagers and adult men and women. In section **9** we look at how you can try to prevent problems and how to treat them if they do happen.

5.8 Babies and children

If a baby is born with sickle cell anaemia, there are usually no signs until after the age of 3 months.

Babies over the age of 3 months and children **may** have **some** of the problems below. Please remember that we have listed all the possibilities; nobody will have all or even most of these.

● Babies and children may sometimes get **painful swollen hands and feet** (hand-foot syndrome). This often happens when a child is between 6 months and 2 years old.

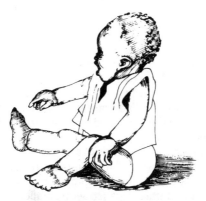

● They may have **painful crises.** These pains, sometimes with swelling and tenderness, may occur in various parts of the body, but most often in the arms and legs. They sometimes cause swollen joints, for example in the knees and elbows. Painful crises can also occur in the back, chest and tummy. The pain may last for only a few hours, or for as long as a week, or even longer. Sometimes the child also has a temperature. (See sections **5.5** and **5.6** on what to do to help someone who has a painful crisis).

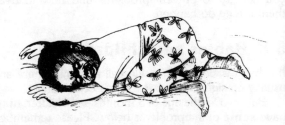

● Babies and children may get **infections**. The most common kinds of infections are pneumonia (infection in the lungs) and malaria (see section **5.4**). Pneumonia usually begins with a cough, a high temperature, and chest pains. Other kinds of infection are also common. Meningitis (infection in the liquid which surrounds the spine and the brain), and septicaemia (blood poisoning) are particularly dangerous. Infections can be very serious. If your child has a high temperature seek medical help immediately.

● Most children with sickle cell disease have **anaemia**, but most of the time this does not cause any problems. A child with anaemia may look pale, have little energy, feel tired and be short of breath.

● Some children may have **splenic sequestration**. The blood in the spleen sickles and the spleen quickly becomes very large. This happens mainly in small children. The child has a tummy ache and may have a high temperature. Splenic sequestration is relatively common in younger children and is very dangerous. Take the child to hospital immediately. In some clinics doctors teach the mothers how to feel for the spleen. This simple test can help the family to recognise this serious complication in its early stages.

● Many children have slightly yellow whites of their eyes. This is called **jaundice** and is caused by the

46

quick destruction of the red blood cells. Yellow whites of the eyes are not unusual for people with sickle cell disease. They do not mean that the child has an infectious illness or something wrong with the liver. However, if the child gets gall stones or has sickling in the liver his or her eyes will turn very yellow, often suddenly. Discuss any sudden changes with your doctor.

● Most children and adults with sickle cell disease need to **pass water many times a day**. This is because their kidneys are slightly affected by the disease. To keep their kidneys as healthy as possible, and to prevent their blood from becoming too thick, which may cause sickling, people with sickle cell disease must always drink plenty of liquid. They will need to pass water more frequently. It is important to explain this to children and to their teachers at school.

● Because they need to drink so much, and have difficulty concentrating their urine, some children may have problems with **bed wetting**. This will go away in time. It is most important that your child should drink as much as possible, so never try to prevent him or her drinking, for example in the evening. Children with bed wetting problems may need comfort and support.

● People with sickle cell disease often have very **dark urine**. This is not dangerous. Sometimes the urine may have blood in it. This usually means that there has been some sickling in the kidney and a blood vessel has burst open and bled. Always tell the doctor if there has been blood in your urine.

● Some children with sickle cell disease may have a **large stomach**, perhaps due to an enlarged spleen.

● Children with sickle cell disease often have **nose-bleeds**, due to sickling in the blood vessels. Although these are troublesome they are not dangerous.

● Sometimes sickle cell disease may make a child's **teeth stick out**. Discuss it with your doctor.

● Children with sickle cell disease often have a **poor**

appetite and do not feel like eating. If you are worried it might help to discuss this with your doctor or staff at the health centre.

● A small number of children with sickle cell disease have **strokes**. These happen when sickled cells block the blood vessels in the brain. Strokes can sometimes cause weakness or paralysis down one side of the body, speech difficulties, loss of memory, or eye problems. We do not know exactly why they happen but they are not common.

These problems may continue as a child grows older, and are also found, though less frequently, in adults. In section **5.9** we look at problems that particularly affect teenagers and adults.

5.9 Teenagers and adults

Teenagers with sickle cell disease may grow more slowly and reach puberty later than other children but they will reach normal adulthood in time.

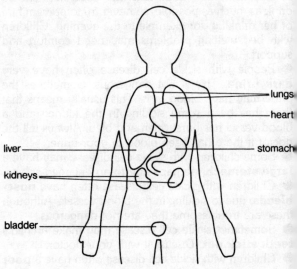

● In certain parts of the world, e.g. Jamaica, people with sickle cell disease often have **sores** and ulcers round their ankles.

● People with sickle cell disease sometimes have **gallstones**. The gall bladder is an organ near the liver. Gallstones can be very painful and can cause jaundice. They sometimes have to be removed by an operation.

● Occasionally people get sickling of the red blood cells in the lung. This is called **chest syndrome**. The person gets a high temperature and pain in the chest with a cough. Chest syndrome should be treated in hospital.

● Sometimes sickling in the blood vessels of the eye can cause **blurred vision** and even **loss of sight**. If you notice any problems with your eyes, inform your doctor. Early treatment may prevent it getting worse.

● People in their 50s and 60s with sickle cell disease disease may develop **kidney disease**. It is wise to get regular check-ups over the age of 40 years.

● Some people with sickle cell disease get **weak bones**. This is because when the red blood cells sickle they often block the blood vessels that feed the bones. This happens most often in the shoulder and hip bones which can become weak and sometimes even damaged. If you have pain in your hips or shoulders tell your doctor.

● Young adults with sickle cell disease may get **peptic ulcers** (stomach ulcers). Once these are recognised they are easy to treat. Always tell your doctor about any stomach pain.

● **Pregnancy**. Women with sickle cell disease conceive normally, and, if they have proper care, usually have a normal pregnancy and healthy children. But pregnancy puts extra stresses on your body. So you may be more likely to have painful crises, infections, malaria, kidney problems and eye problems caused by sickling while you are pregnant, so you need extra care and attention. **If you are preg-**

nant, tell your doctor as soon as possible. He or she will want to keep a special eye on you throughout your pregnancy to make sure you stay well.

● Teenage boys and men may suffer from **priapism**. This is a painful erection of the penis caused by sickling of the blood vessels. Priapism is extremely painful and you should see a doctor as soon as possible. Continued priapism for several days may lead to impotence.

Priapism may be caused or made worse if your bladder is full and pressing on your private parts. When an attack begins empty your bladder immediately. Take a cold shower or put a cold compress on your penis. Take some exercise to get your blood circulating – a quick run, or a few pull-ups or sit-ups. If it does not settle in 6 hours, go to the hospital but also report each episode at the clinic.

You may prevent priapism by making sure that you drink plenty of liquid and pass water as often as possible, getting up during the night if necessary. A note from a young man with sickle cell disease:

'Recently I have been getting painful attacks of priapism. I wake up in the early morning with a painful erection. This starts with a small burning sensation in my penis. The pain quickly grows more intense until it becomes unbearable.

I have found that a 'crisis' is often caused by tension in my penis and anus. This usually happens when my bowels and bladder are not completely empty, so a visit to the toilet will often help it to subside quicker. I have found that it is better to get up and exercise, go for short walks, rather than to lie down and try to ignore it. I have found the erection to be the main cause, so once that goes the pain goes.

Like myself, many male sufferers are embarrassed to talk about their private problems, especially to female doctors. Male sufferers may be happier to talk openly to other men with sickle cell disease or to male doctors.'

● **Anaesthetics**. Gases or drugs used before an operation to put people to sleep. The effects of anaesthetics on the body may lead to sickling. People with sickle cell disease can still have anaesthetics but must tell doctors, dentists, or nurses that they have sickle cell disease, so that special care can be taken.

PLEASE REMEMBER THAT MOST PEOPLE WITH SICKLE CELL ANAEMIA AND OTHER KINDS OF SICKLE CELL DISEASE HAVE ONLY **SOME** OF THE PROBLEMS WE HAVE LISTED ABOVE.

⑥ SC disease (Hb SC)

SC disease occurs when a child inherits sickle haemo-globin (Hb S) from one parent and haemoglobin C (Hb C) from the other. It is not as common at birth as sickle cell anaemia, and it generally causes milder problems.

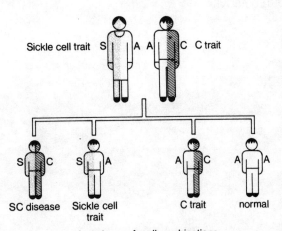

1 in 4 chance for all combinations

Haemoglobin C is thought to originate in West Africa. It is found in 1 out of every 5 inhabitants (20%) of northern Ghana and is also common in the Ivory Coast. It is also found among people living in western Nigeria, Sierra Leone and Liberia but here the incidence is much lower. Descendants of these people living in America, the West Indies and Britain also carry haemoglobin C gene. It is occasionally found in North Africa and the Mediterranean.

Persons with SC disease are usually less anaemic

than those with sickle cell anaemia. In fact, their haemoglobin level may be in the normal range. This has its advantages and disadvantages. On the whole, they tend to have fewer crises and suffer less severe infections such as pneumonia. On the other hand, because of the high haemoglobin, their blood is thicker than those with sickle cell anaemia, and this makes them more likely to have problems in the small vessels of the eye. Occasionally sickling in the eye can cause partial or total loss of vision. The joint problems are often confused with rheumatism, as these affect the joints of the hips and shoulders.

Other problems are similar to those found in sickle cell anaemia. Management of SC disease is the same as sickle cell anaemia. It is essential that a person with SC disease drinks enough fluid, takes folic acid and antimalarial tablets. Some doctors may also prescribe penicillin to prevent infection. Pregnant women must be seen by a doctor, so that their pregnancy and childbirth can be supervised.

(7) Sickle beta-thalassaemia (Hb S Beta-thal)

(Please read section **5** as well.)

Sickle beta-thalassaemia (Hb S Beta-thal) occurs when a child inherits sickle haemoglobin (Hb S) from one parent and thalassaemia (Beta-thal) from the other.

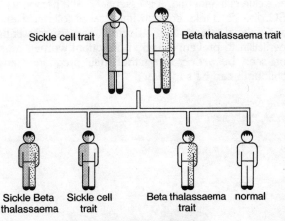

Sickle cell trait   Beta thalassaema trait

Sickle Beta   Sickle cell   Beta thalassaema   normal
thalassaema   trait   trait

1 in 4 chance for all combinations

A person who has inherited thalassaemia cannot make as much haemoglobin as normal. A person with one thalassaemia gene and one sickle haemoglobin gene may sometimes get sickling of the red blood cells.

There are two kinds of sickle beta-thalassaemia. A special test can tell you which kind you have.

1 If someone has **sickle beta°-thalassaemia** (Hb S Beta°-thal) their red blood cells contain only sickle haemoglobin (Hb S). The symptoms of sickle beta°-thalassaemia are similar to those of sickle cell anaemia (see section **5**).

2 **sickle beta⁺-thalassaemia** (Hb S Beta⁺-thal) is not so serious; the symptoms are similar to those of SC disease (see section **6**). In sickle beta⁺-thalassaemia the red blood cells contain mainly sickle haemoglobin (Hb S) and some normal haemoglobin, haemoglobin A.

If you have either kind of sickle beta-thalassaemia it is **very** important to tell the doctor **before** you have an anaesthetic and **as soon as** you are pregnant so that extra care can be taken to keep you well.

To find out more about thalassaemia ask your doctor or contact the U.K. Thalassaemia Society, 107 Nightingale Road, London N8.

⑧ Testing for sickle cell disease

8.1 Blood tests

There are several special blood tests which can show whether a person has sickle cell disease or sickle cell trait. It is possible to test new born babies as well as adults. It is also possible to test babies before they are born (see section **8.2**).

There are three main tests:
1 The sickle test
2 The solubility test
3 Haemoglobin electrophoresis

1 The Sickle or Sickling Test This test shows whether you have sickle haemoglobin in your blood. It only requires one drop of blood mixed with a reducing agent on a glass slide covered by a smaller piece of glass and sealed so that oxygen does not reach the red blood cells in the drop. The test does not distinguish between sickle cell disease and sickle cell trait. Also, it **cannot** be used to test

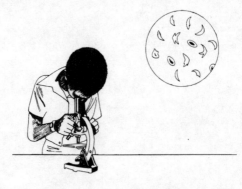

babies under one year old, as the results are not reliable. All young babies should be tested by haemoglobin electrophoresis.

2 The Solubility Test This test depends on the fact that haemoglobin S is less soluble (dissolves less easily) than haemoglobin A when mixed with certain chemicals in small glass tubes. It can serve as a guide in distinguishing between sickle cell anaemia, sickle cell trait and the normal haemoglobin (Hb A). But it has similar drawbacks to the sickling test, and haemoglobin electrophoresis must be carried out to confirm the result.

3 Haemoglobin Electrophoresis This is the most important test for sickle cell disease. It tells you exactly what kind of haemoglobin you have, for example Hb SS, Hb AS or Hb AC. There are some types of haemoglobin that give a similar result in this test, for example haemoglobin S and haemoglobin D. However, by changing the type of chemicals used in the test, most of these haemoglobin types can be distinguished from one another. The sickle and solubility tests can sometimes help to separate one from the other when used with haemoglobin electrophoresis.

With the sickle test, the result is either 'sickle positive' or 'sickle negative'. 'Sickle positive' shows that you have either sickle cell trait or sickle cell disease. It cannot show which. 'Sickle negative' only shows that there is no sickle haemoglobin (Hb S) in your blood. It does not say what kind of haemoglobin you have. For example, a person with C trait (Hb AC) or thalassaemia trait (Hb A Beta-thal) would have a 'sickle negative' result. You need a haemoglobin electrophoresis test to see if you have C trait and other laboratory tests to see if you have thalassaemia trait.

However it is still important to carry out sickle tests as some haemoglobins may look like S on haemoglobin electrophoresis, such as D, but do not sickle.

If you have already been to your doctor for a blood test, and you were only given the result 'sickle positive' or 'sickle negative' ask for the results of your haemoglobin electrophoresis test.

8.2 Testing babies before they are born

It is now possible to test babies for sickle cell disease while they are still in their mother's womb. If the baby is found to have sickle cell disease the parents may decide that they want to terminate the pregnancy.

THERE ARE THREE TESTS:
1 Chorionic Villi Sampling
Chorionic villi are finger-like projections that initially surround the unborn baby and attach it to the inside surface of the womb. They subsequently develop into the placenta (after birth). Doctors are now able to take a small piece of the villi, and use them in the laboratory for testing for sickle cell disease. The advantage of this method is that it can be done between the 8th and 11th week of pregnancy.

2 Amniotic Fluid Sampling
Doctors take a small amount of the liquid surrounding the baby in the mother's womb to find out what kind of haemoglobin it has. For medical reasons this test will only work if both parent's blood is a special type, so both parents will need to have a blood test first.

3 Fetal Blood Sampling
This test is not commonly undertaken now. Doctors take a drop of the unborn baby's blood after the third month of pregnancy through a special tube inserted into the womb. The blood is tested in the laboratory to find out what kind of haemoglobin the baby has.

The last two tests can only be done later on in the

pregnancy, after three months (16 – 20 weeks). This can increase the risk of complications and abortion. All the three tests can sometimes cause miscarriage through disturbing the unborn baby.

At the moment these tests can only be done in a few hospitals; mostly in Europe, the United States and Australia. It is important to emphasise that the decision to undergo these tests and to terminate an affected pregnancy is entirely that of the couple. Doctors and health workers can only help by discussing with them the various methods and likely complications that can occur, and then allow them to decide whether they would like to have the test. The couple can then inform their doctor who will help to establish contact with any of the centres where the tests are done, if they want one.

For further information please contact the nearest society/centre listed in section **12**.

⑨ Looking after somebody with sickle cell disease

As yet there is no cure for sickle cell disease. A person who is born with sickle cell disease will have it for the rest of their life. However, we are now able to prevent some of the problems that people used to have.

Here is a list of practical hints that people have given us which may help someone with sickle cell disease stay as healthy as possible. We have written this section especially for people with sickle cell disease, but it may also be helpful to parents and friends and other people who are close to them.

9.1 General medical care

● It is important to know exactly what kind of sickle cell disease you have. You can have a test to find out (see section **8.1**). It is also important that **whenever you are ill or have an accident or need any medical or dental treatment** you always tell the doctors and nurses that you have sickle cell disease and what kind you have.

Some hospitals give you a card which states what kind of sickle cell disease you have. You can carry this round with you and show it in emergencies.

● If you have sickle cell disease you should have regular check-ups at the hospital. Discuss with your doctor how often these should be. Don't miss these check-ups even if you are feeling well. Doctors need to know how you are when you are well so that they know your normal state. Medical tests can also often pick up problems at a very early stage, even before you are aware of them. Early treatment may prevent later problems. Some people have had problems getting the medical help and advice they need. If you are having any difficulty please contact the nearest Society/Centre listed in section **12**.

● Do not be frightened or embarrassed to talk to your doctor about any problems or worries you have. Parents, friends and relatives may also want to talk to someone about their worries and fears. Most doctors are happy to help.

● The treatment that doctors give varies a lot. Doctors have different ideas about how best to treat sickle cell disease. All are agreed on the need to prevent malaria. It is **vital** to take regular anti-malarial medicine. Always ask doctors and nurses to discuss with you what they are doing and why. It is most important that you should understand and feel confident about all the treatment you have. Some doctors prescribe daily penicillin syrup or tablets to prevent infections. Some doctors prescribe folic acid tablets; these help your body make red blood cells.

You may sometimes need **blood transfusions**. Here are some of the reasons why doctors may advise one.

● If you are having a very severe crisis which is taking a long time to get better the doctors may decide that a transfusion will stop the crisis more quickly.

● If you have become very anaemic either because of malaria, or because your spleen is enlarged, or you just cannot make enough blood for the time being the transfusion will bring your blood back to normal and give you time to recover.

● If you need an operation, for example a tonsillectomy (taking out the tonsils) or a splenectomy (taking out the spleen).

● If you have had a stroke you may be given a transfusion every 4 to 6 weeks for about 3 years. This prevents further strokes and helps you to recover.

You may be given an **exchange transfusion**. This means that the doctor first takes some sickle blood from you and then gives you normal donor blood. This is repeated until you have almost no sickle blood left. Exchange transfusion is the safest kind of transfusion because it leaves little sickle blood in the circulation and also because you are not left with extra iron from the extra blood.

Always ask your doctor to explain exactly why you are having a transfusion.

● Make sure that you and your children with sickle cell disease have been fully immunised against all childhood infections: polio, whooping cough, tetanus, diphtheria, measles, German measles. This is important even if you are taking penicillin.

● If you live in a tropical country, for example Nigeria, you must take protection against malaria. If you are going to visit a tropical area tell your doctor where you are going and ask what kind of anti-malarial medicine you should take. Begin taking it 2 weeks before you go, take it the whole time you are there, and continue for 4 to 6 weeks after you leave the malarial area.

● Do not take any iron pills or tonics. These will not do you any good and they may actually harm you. Your doctor will prescribe any iron or other medicines if you need them.

● You may be tempted to buy potions that are claimed to cure sickle cell disease. At the moment there is no such known cure.

9.2 Care at home

● Always drink plenty of liquids, for example, water milk, fruit juice or squash. This is particularly important if you are feeling ill. If you do not have enough liquid in your body you become dehydrated. Your blood gets thicker and your red blood cells stick together. This could cause sickling. Drink a lot of liquid to help prevent sickling.

● Learn to take your own temperature. If it is over 38° Centigrade or 100.4° Fahrenheit seek medical advice.

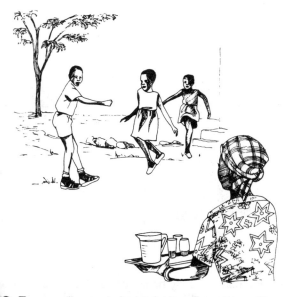

● Too much exercise may make you tired and bring on pain. Everybody needs some exercise to keep fit, so don't stop altogether. Learn how much your body can take and make sure you don't overdo it.
● If you are at school, college or work, make sure that the people there know that you have sickle cell disease and what you can and cannot do. If they don't know very much, give them this guide to read.
● Up to now no special food has been found which will help people with sickle cell disease. Just eat a healthy diet, with as much fruit and vegetables as you can.
● You will probably worry about pain, about going to hospital, and even about the possibility of dying at an early age. It is very important that you are able to

talk freely to someone about this. If you want help and advice ask someone you like and trust, for example your doctor, a health worker, or a friend.

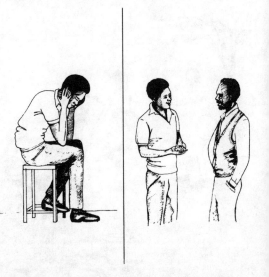

● Although you may be ill from time to time, try not to think of yourself as a permanent invalid. When you are well, try to live as normal a life as possible. Keep an eye on your health but don't let sickle cell disease take over your whole life.

⑩ How sickle cell disease may affect families

This section is particularly for parents who have found out that their child has sickle cell disease but we hope that it will be useful to everybody.

When parents are told that their child has inherited sickle cell disease, they often feel shocked, guilty, angry, frightened, and very distressed. These are perfectly normal and natural feelings. But we have found that as parents learn more about their child's condition, these feelings begin to go away, and most parents feel more confident about managing. Below are some of the most common feelings that parents and other family members have mentioned to us.

SHOCK OR DENIAL 'It must be a mistake. . . . It can't be true.'

This is a perfectly natural reaction, particularly if neither of you has a history of the illness in your family.

GUILT 'It's my fault. . . . I must have done something to cause this.'

Parents often regard their child's illness as a punishment for something they have done. Brothers and sisters may also feel guilty because they are healthy and cannot 'take their share' of the pain. Try to overcome any guilt you feel. It doesn't help the child and it doesn't help you. In fact, guilt can do a lot of harm in families. The whole family needs to be reassured that the illness is nobody's fault.

BLAME 'It's your fault. . . . You must have done something to cause this.'

It is quite common for one partner to blame the other, or to think that it must be his or her side of the family which is passing on the illness. People may say things like 'Nobody in our family has ever had this illness before, so it must be from your side.' This is unfair. Sickle cell disease is nobody's 'fault'. In fact, sickle cell disease must be inherited from **both** parents.

There will be times when children blame their parents because they have sickle cell disease. This can be very hurtful, particularly when you have given so much to your child. But remember that people who are in any kind of pain and suffering often turn their anger and unhappiness on those they love most.

ANGER 'It's not fair.'

Parents are often angry, because there are so many things to be angry about. For example, you cannot predict when a child with sickle cell disease will become ill, so it is often difficult to plan ahead. A family may have to change its lifestyle to fit in with the child. This may cause a lot of anger or resentment. Family members may angrily blame the affected child for 'causing' these changes. Or they may direct the blame at someone else in the family. There may be tension and rows.

Parents may also feel angry towards doctors and nurses. As well as the shock of learning that their child has sickle cell disease, they may feel uncomfortable and ill at ease in a hospital or with medical people. They may feel that doctors and nurses have not been as helpful or caring as they could have been. They may be so upset that they cannot fully understand what the doctors and nurses are telling them. Many parents have complained to us that they did not get the information they wanted in a way that they could easily understand. This guide was written to help with this problem.

FEAR 'I'm so afraid. . . . I can't cope.'

Parents are naturally frightened about whether they will be able to cope and if their child will die at an early age. They may be very anxious about what will happen if they have more affected children. Also, many people are scared of doctors, and are naturally frightened of looking stupid or of not understanding what they have been told. Some parents find it easier to talk about their fears to other parents who have children with sickle cell disease.

HELPLESSNESS 'It's terrible to feel we can't do anything. . . . I can't manage.'

When your child is ill and in pain, particularly during a painful crisis, you may quite naturally feel that you would much rather suffer the pain yourself. You may feel bad that you cannot stop the pain for your child. But although you may not always be able to take the pain away, there are other practical ways in which you can help your child at times like this. (See sections **5.5** and **5.6** on dealing with a painful crisis). Your support and love will help your child greatly.

SHAME 'How can we tell our friends? . . . I don't want anybody to know.'

Until recently, there was very little real information about sickle cell disease. There were a lot of myths and misleading or incorrect statements which caused parents a great deal of distress. Sickle cell disease is still viewed by some people in our community as a dreadful and shameful illness which mainly affects black people. This fact alone can create stigma. Because of it families often feel acutely embarrassed about having an affected child. It is important to know that similar inherited conditions exist in other ethnic groups, for example, cystic fibrosis in white people, and tay-sachs disease in European Jews. The more we educate people about sickle cell disease the less shame and embarrassment there will be. Most people will support and help you, not blame you.

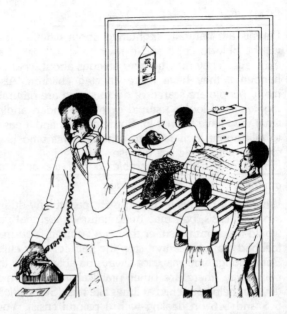

IT IS A CURSE 'Somebody does not like my family and is cursing us.'

Sickle cell disease is not a curse on any family and nobody can put a curse on anybody else: it is an inherited disease. So do not let ill feelings spoil your relationship with your neighbours or relations. You may need their help and support in time of crises.

JEALOUSY FROM BROTHERS AND SISTERS 'You love him more than me.'

Healthy brothers and sisters may be jealous because they do not get as much attention as they would like. Your partner may also feel neglected, because you are devoting all your time to your sick child. It might help to discuss these feelings. Or you may find that there are things you can do to make the rest of the family less jealous. The whole family needs to be involved in looking after a child with sickle cell disease.

68

JEALOUSY FROM THE CHILD 'Why aren't I the same as you?'

The whole family needs to be aware that a child with sickle cell disease may be jealous because he or she is not blessed with good health like his or her brothers or sisters.

The more information that you all have about sickle cell disease, the better. **Every member of the family** has to adjust emotionally to the child's illness, and each person must come to terms with it in his or her own way. Everyone will need to talk about their feelings, so it is important to create opportunities for this. If you would like more advice or help, contact your doctor, social worker, health visitor, church minister, or your local sickle cell group.

⑪ Questions that people often ask about sickle cell disease

1 *When was sickle cell disease first discovered?*

Sickle shaped cells were first reported in 1910 by Dr Herrick in Chicago. He found them when he was examining the blood of a West Indian student who complained of tiredness and pains in the body. Looking through a microscope Dr Herrick found that some of the red blood cells had an unusual sickle shape instead of the normal round one.

2 *Will my child grow out of sickle cell disease?*

No, because it is an inherited illness. This means that your child will have it for the rest of his or her life. However, most people do not have the symptoms of sickle cell disease all the time. They may go for several months, or even years, without any problems. This sometimes makes parents think that their child no longer has the illness, but the symptoms can come back any time. In general, adults seem to have less pain than children or teenagers.

3 *How long do people with sickle cell disease usually live?*

There is no simple answer to this question. Some people live to a ripe old age and some die young. There are many elderly people alive and well with sickle cell disease. Some people suffer a lot of pain and illness, while others lead almost normal lives.

Every individual is different. There are also different kinds of sickle cell disease, some of which are quite mild, and even among people with the same kind of sickle cell disease, there are great variations in their symptoms.

4 Is there a cure for sickle cell disease?

No, there is no cure for sickle cell disease at present. If a person is born with it they will have it for the rest of their life.

5 Are there any herbs that can cure sickle cell disease?

No. At this point in time, no herbs have been found to cure sickle cell disease. However, several people have claimed that they have discovered herbal preparations that can cure sickle cell disease. This is difficult to prove since sickle cell disease is quite variable in severity and frequency of crises. Whereas some individuals have a very mild and uneventful course, others have severe problems frequently. Even in the last group, the problems may only occur every so often. People can therefore claim success in curing the disease while in fact the improvement may have occurred as a result of the natural course of the illness.

There are research centres, for example in Nigeria, trying to test some of these herbs, and to find out whether they are harmful to any part of the body. Only then can such herbs be claimed to have any effect on sickle cell disease.

6 I have sickle cell disease. Can I have children?

Yes. However, women with sickle cell disease need special care during pregnancy. When a woman is pregnant the changes in her body may cause her blood to sickle. Women with sickle cell disease also have a higher risk of miscarriages. Because of these extra risks it is most important to think carefully about becoming pregnant and to

71

tell your doctor as soon as you are pregnant (see section **5.9**).

Men with sickle cell disease can certainly become fathers. But it is known that some men who have had priapism (a painful erection; pain in the private parts due to sickling) sometimes become impotent, and may have difficulty fathering children (see section **5.9**). However, specialist advice is available which may help.

7 *If a person has sickle cell disease, will their children have it?*

This depends on what kind of haemoglobin their partner has. For example, if they have sickle cell anaemia (Hb SS) and their partner has the usual haemoglobin (Hb AA), all their children will be born with sickle cell trait (Hb AS). None of them will have sickle cell anaemia.

But, if they have sickle cell anaemia (Hb SS) and their partner has sickle cell trait (Hb AS), there is a 1 in 2 (50%) chance that each child will have either sickle cell anaemia (Hb SS) or sickle cell trait (Hb AS).

Finally, if both they and their partner have sickle cell anaemia (Hb SS) all their children will have sickle cell anaemia (Hb SS). (For more about inheritance see section **4**.)

8 *Do only black people get sickle cell disease?*

No. Sickle cell disease is found in people whose families originated in all those parts of the world where there is malaria, for example, Africa, the Middle East, Asia and some countries in the Mediterranean area such as Turkey and Greece (see the map on page 22). Sickle cell trait seems to offer some protection against malaria.

9 *Is sickle cell disease only passed on by women?*

No. The genes for sickle cell disease can be passed on by both men and women.

10 *Do boys get sickle cell disease more often than girls?*

No. It is found equally among both boys and girls.

11 *My daughter has sickle cell trait, should her partner be tested?*

Yes, if they want to know whether there is a risk of having a child with sickle cell disease. If your daughter's partner also has a trait there is then a 1 in 4 (25%) chance that each child will inherit sickle cell disease.

12 *I have had many blood tests in the past. Surely I would have been told by now if I had sickle cell trait?*

Not necessarily, for several reasons. Firstly, doctors have to do a special blood test to find out whether you have sickle haemoglobin in your blood. Secondly, even if they do the test, because sickle cell trait is not an illness, doctors do not always tell people that they have it. Ask if you can have a haemoglobin electrophoresis test (see section **8.1**) and ask the doctor to tell you the result, whatever it is.

13 *I have been told I am 'sickle positive'. What does that mean?*

'Sickle positive' means that you have sickle haemoglobin in your blood. It does not tell you whether you have sickle cell trait or a kind of sickle cell disease. You need to have a haemoglobin electrophoresis test (see section **8.1**) to tell you which you have.

14 *Why do some people with sickle cell disease suffer more pain than others?*

Sadly, nobody really knows, not even the medical experts. But here are some possible reasons:

Firstly, there are different kinds of sickle cell

disease, and some are more severe than others. For example, SC disease and one kind of sickle beta-thalassaemia are usually less severe than sickle cell anaemia. Also, some people with sickle cell disease inherit other genes as well, such as alpha-thalassaemia or fetal haemoglobin, which make the effects of sickle cell disease milder.

Secondly, sickle cell disease affects people differently at different ages. For example, young children under the age of 5 may have pain and infections quite frequently. They then often have very few symptoms for several years. When they become teenagers they may start to have problems again until they reach adulthood. Every person has a different pattern.

Thirdly, the effects of sickle cell disease are made worse if people have poor housing or a poor diet or if they have difficulty getting good medical care. We also believe that if families understand more about sickle cell disease they can cope much better.

15 *Are there any particular times of the year when crises are more common?*

Crises can occur at any time of the year, but in the tropical areas where there are mainly two seasons — wet and dry — problems are commoner when it is cold and dry, such as during the harmattan (cold, dusty and windy) season in West Africa. Also, during the hot, rainy season, over exposure and unnecessary exertion can lead to dehydration and cause crises. Even in the cooler climates, crises tend to occur more frequently during the cold winter months.

It is therefore important to adjust the clothing to suit the varying weather conditions to avoid crises. Do not allow persons having sickle cell disease to get exposed to extremes of cold and hot weather.

16 *Is there any research going on into sickle cell disease?*

Yes. We know about people doing research in America, Jamaica, Britain and Africa into several different areas. Here are some of them:

● Some researchers are trying to find anti-sickling drugs which would stop the red blood cells from sickling. They have found several chemicals that can do this but unfortunately, so far, they all have serious side effects and make people ill. Researchers are now trying to reduce these side effects so that the drug can be given safely. Anti-sickling drugs could be used to prevent or relieve painful crises. They would also prevent the other problems that sickling causes.

● Some people are looking into the possibility of treatment with bone marrow transplants. These would stop a person producing sickle haemoglobin. However, even though this treatment is used occasionally for patients with some blood conditions, it is still experimental.

● Some people are researching into genetic engineering, but this is also still in the experimental stage. They are trying to alter the haemoglobin genes so that a person who has inherited sickle cell disease could still produce normal haemoglobin.

● Other people are looking into different aspects of sickle cell disease such as pain, problems with the spleen, and protection against infections.

17 *We already have one child with sickle cell disease. Can we do anything to prevent another child being born with the disease?*

There are two ways of preventing the birth of a child with sickle cell disease. *Either* you can decide not to have any more children at all, in case one of them has sickle cell disease; *or*, if you want to try for another child, you can now test the baby

75

before it is born to see if it has sickle cell disease. If the result shows that the baby has sickle cell disease you may then decide to terminate (end) the pregnancy. Only a few centres in Europe, the United States of America and Australia can carry out this test. If you need more help contact the nearest organisation listed in section **12**.

18 *We both have sickle cell trait. Will all our children be born with sickle cell anaemia?*

Not necessarily. If you read the section on inheritance, (section **4**) you will see that if both parents have a trait there are several possibilities for their children. It is just a matter of chance what kind of haemoglobin each child inherits. This is why, in the same family, there are often children with sickle cell anaemia, children with sickle cell trait and children with normal haemoglobin.

If both parents have sickle cell trait each child can have either the disease, or the trait, or normal haemoglobin. Each child has the same chances. So, it is possible that all your children might have sickle cell anaemia, or sickle cell trait, or normal haemoglobin, or, each child may have a different haemoglobin. It's all a matter of chance.

19 *I have been told that my baby girl has sickle cell disease. When should I expect the problems to start?*

Problems do not usually start until the baby is 3 months old. Until then she will have mainly fetal haemoglobin (Hb F). We all have this fetal haemoglobin when we are born and it gradually disappears between 3 and 4 months. Then your baby will have mainly sickle haemoglobin and so her red blood cells may begin to sickle. However, some babies with sickle cell disease have no problems till they are 1 or 2 years old, or even older.

20 *I have four children living in the same room. One of them has sickle cell disease and the others have either normal haemoglobin or sickle cell trait. Can his disease be transferred to any of them through insect bites, in the way that malaria is transferred by mosquito bites?*

No. There is no possibility of transfer of sickle cell anaemia by insect bites. Therefore your other children will not catch the illness. Sickle cell disease is not an infection like malaria as has been pointed out earlier. (See section **2**).

21 *My child does not eat very much. What can I do?*

Many parents of children with sickle cell disease have found that their children have a poor appetite. It is obviously important to try and encourage your child to eat a good diet, but if people make too much fuss mealtimes could become a battleground. Children with sickle cell disease tend to be thin. This is not necessarily related to how much they eat.

22 *Is there any special food you should eat if you have sickle cell disease?*

It is important to eat a good healthy, balanced diet, but up to now nobody has found any particular food that helps people with sickle cell disease. Since sickle cell disease is not caused by a lack of iron in the diet, it is not necessary, and it may be harmful to take tonics that contain iron.

23 *Can I give my child who has sickle cell disease immunisation against infections?*

Yes. It is very important to get your child with sickle cell disease immunised against infections. It is known that such children are more likely to get infections and therefore need help to fight conditions such as measles, tetanus, poliomyelitis, etc. In fact some doctors give regular penicillin medicine to all children with sickle cell anaemia to help prevent infection. Immunisation is one of the most effective ways of preventing infections. Contact your doctor or health officer for more information about immunisation.

24 My child wets the bed a lot. Is this because he has sickle cell disease?

Yes, it could be. We know that children with sickle cell disease are more likely to wet their beds for longer than other children. They will grow out of it in the end but meanwhile you might discuss this problem with your doctor or local clinic. They may be able to help. Even if you are trying to stop the bed-wetting it is very important that you do not cut down the amount of liquid that your child drinks. Children with sickle cell disease should drink plenty of liquid to help prevent their blood sickling (see section **5.8**). It is important to remember that children with bed-wetting problems will need comfort and support.

25 Will sickle cell disease cripple my child?

Most children and adults with sickle cell disease live very reasonable lives. Looking at them nobody can tell that they have the disease. However, a very few people have strokes due to sickling in the brain. This can cause problems with walking and speech. Sickling in the blood vessels of the bones in the hip may sometimes make movement difficult and can cause a limp. Finally a few people have sickling of the blood vessels in the eye and this can lead to loss of sight in one or both eyes. But please remember that most people with sickle cell disease are **not** disabled in these ways, and that many problems can be prevented with regular hospital care.

26 *My teenage daughter has sickle cell disease and I am worried about her periods and whether she will have problems.*

We know that girls with sickle cell disease may start their periods a few years later than other girls. Some girls may have severe pain and cramps just before or during periods. These may lead to a crisis. Please discuss this with your doctor who may prescribe painkillers.

27 *My daughter has sickle cell disease and wants to go on the pill. Is it safe for her?*

Doctors have different opinions about this. Medical experts feel that it is safer to prescribe the kind of pill that contains only progesterone. Other birth control methods, such as the cap, certainly wouldn't cause any problems. She should definitely make sure that her doctor or family planning clinic knows that she has sickle cell disease.

28 *Will sickle cell disease affect my child's education?*

Sickle cell disease does not affect the mental ability of a child, except very occasionally if a child has a stroke. However, problems may arise if your child is away from school a lot through illness. It is very important that you and your child's teachers do everything you can to prevent problems. For example, if your child is away from school special help may be needed with catching up on the missed work.

If you feel that your child's education is suffering because of frequent illnesses, please discuss this with his or her teachers. It may be possible to arrange for the child to be taught at home if he has to stay at home in bed.

29 *Are there any sports that my daughter should not do because she has sickle cell disease?*

Children with sickle cell disease should be encouraged to take part in sport and to find out how much they can manage. This will vary from child to child. For example, some children can go swimming, and others can not. Very tiring exercise, such as cross-country running, may be too difficult for a child with sickle cell disease. Sports such as deep sea diving, which can lower the level of oxygen in the body, may cause problems. Sports involving holding the breath, such as underwater swimming, should be avoided. It is important after swimming or showering, not to get cold and to dry well and wrap up warmly. This advice also applies to those areas in the tropics where children may often swim in streams, ponds and rivers.

The most important point is that each child is different and it is up to the child and its parents to find out how much he or she can tolerate. It is important to treat children with sickle cell disease as normally as possible and not to be too overprotective. On the other hand, children should not be forced to take part in a strenuous sporting activity if they feel that it will bring on a painful crisis or breathlessness.

30 *Are there any jobs or careers that a child with sickle cell disease should not aim for?*

People with sickle cell disease can do almost any job. Very strenuous work or work outdoors in all types of weather would probably not be suitable. You should discuss the question of careers with your child as early as possible and in a positive way. Don't just mention the jobs your child should not do but give him or her examples of people with sickle cell disease who have been successful in different careers. For example, in the reading list in section **13** we give details of an article written by a successful doctor, Joseph Phillips, who has sickle cell anaemia. Examples like this will give children confidence that, despite their health problems, they can be successful in most fields.

31 *I have read that it is dangerous for people with sickle cell disease to fly. Is this true?*

Not necessarily. Many people who have sickle cell disease fly all over the world, for example to the West Indies and Africa, without any problems. Nevertheless we know that a reduced supply of oxygen and dehydration can cause sickling and this sometimes happens when flying. Long tiring journeys and lack of exercise can also cause problems. If you plan to fly discuss it with your doctor.

Here is some simple practical advice:

● Before and during the flight, drink plenty of liquid, such as water or fruit juice, so that you don't get dehydrated.
● When you can, take some exercise by occasionally walking up and down the aisle of the plane. This will encourage the blood to circulate in your body and reduce the possibility of sickling due to staying in one position for too long.

32 *Why do doctors sometimes advise against blood transfusions? Surely blood transfusions would stop the symptoms of sickle cell disease?*

This is true but blood transfusions can sometimes cause extra problems. For example, if a person has too many blood transfusions they may get too much iron in the blood and this may harm the heart or the liver. Also people may get an allergic reaction to the blood.

At the same time, blood transfusions can sometimes be very helpful (see section **9.1**). If your doctor advises one, always ask him or her to explain why, so that you can feel confident and well informed.

33 *If I have sickle cell trait can I give blood?*

Yes, there is no reason why you cannot donate blood.

34 *Why do I have a drip when I go to hospital?*

It is very important to make sure that you have enough liquid in your body to prevent the red blood cells sickling or getting worse. If you are ill you may not be able to drink as much liquid as you need. A drip is the quickest way to get enough liquid into your body.

35 *My uncle insists that my son, who has sickle cell disease, must have scarification marks over his chest in order to cure the disease. Is this recommended?*

No. Scarification marks do not cure sickle cell disease. They are usually performed over areas of visible pulsations of the heart with the belief that they will cure any concurrent ailment. These pulsations are usually seen in people with fever, anaemia or after physical exercise. It is not unusual therefore for persons with sickle cell disease to have them. Scarification marks will only provide a source of infection which may lead to sickle crises and even death.

⑫ Some useful addresses

The Sickle Cell Society
54 Station Road
Harlesdon
London NW10 4VA
Tel: 081–961–7795

For Thalassaemia:
The United Kingdom Thalassaemia Society
107 Nightingale Lane
London N8
Tel: 081–348–0437

The Caribbean:
Prof. G. Serjeant
Medical Director
Medical Research Council Laboratories
University of the West Indies
Kingston 7
Jamaica
Tel: (809) 927–0687

Nigeria:
Professor Olu Akinyanju
Sickle Cell Club of Nigeria
Department of Medicine
University of Lagos
P.M.B. 12003
Lagos
Nigeria

U.S.A.:
National Association for
Sickle Cell Disease Inc.,
3460 Wilshire Boulevard
Suite 1012
Los Angeles
California 90010–2273
U.S.A.

(13) Further reading about sickle cell disease

Available from the Sickle Cell Society:
(Please send money with your order and enclose a large stamped addressed envelope.)

Sickle Cell Anaemia, Sickle Cell Trait – Booklet Free
Sickle Cell Society 1987

Pain in Sickle Cell Disease, Sickle Cell Society 1986 (£5.95)

Living with Sickle Cell Disease, 1986 (£3.60)

Other publications:
(Your library will be able to order these for you.)

Phillips, Dr. Joseph R. *'How I Cope with Sickle Cell Anaemia'*
Ebony Magazine February 1976

Anionwu, Elizabeth and Beattie, Alan, *'Learning to Cope with Sickle Cell Disease — A Patient's Experience'*
Nursing Times 8 July 1981

Fleming, A. F., ed. *Sickle Cell Disease: A Handbook for the General Clinician*
Churchill Livingstone 1982

Lehmann, H., Huntsman, R. G., *Man's Haemoglobins*
North Holland, Amsterdam 1974

Prashar, U., Anionwu, E., Brozovič, M., *Sickle Cell Anaemia — Who Cares?* Runnymede Trust 1985

Serjeant, G. R., *Sickle Cell Disease*, OUP 1985

(14) Glossary of medical words used in this guide

Below are simple explanations of some of the medical words used in this guide.

Anaesthetics Gases or drugs used before an operation to put people to sleep.

Amniocentesis Withdrawal of the liquid in the mother's womb for testing to find out if her unborn baby is healthy (see section **8.2**).

β The Greek letter B In this guide we have used the English spelling beta, for example, beta-thalassaemia.

Beta-thalassaemia (Beta-thal) Thalassaemia is a condition in which people cannot make enough haemoglobin. There are many kinds of thalassaemia, one of which is beta-thalassaemia (see section **7**).

Blood vessels Very small tubes in the body through which the blood travels (see section **3.4**).

C trait (Hb AC) Someone with C trait has mainly normal haemoglobin but carries the gene for haemoglobin C and could pass it on to their children (see section **4.4**).

Carrier Someone with a trait, that is, one gene for normal haemoglobin and one for another kind. A carrier does not have the disease but 'carries' a gene for it and could pass it on to their children (see section **4.4**).

Chorionic villi Finger like projections that initially surround the unborn baby, from which it is possible to test for sickle cell disease, (see section **8.2**).

Convulsion A fit (see section **5.4**).

Dehydration Not enough water in the body (see section **5.3**).

Fetal blood A baby still in the womb is called a fetus. Fetal blood is the blood the baby has before it is born and for the first three to six months of its life (see section **8.2** and section **11** question 16).

Genes Substances in the mother's egg and the father's sperm through which their characteristics are passed on to the child (see section **4.1**).

Haemoglobin A substance in the red blood cells that carries oxygen round the body. It can also be written as Hb (see section **3**.)

Haemoglobin A (Hb A) Normal adult haemoglobin (see sections **3.3, 4.2** and **4.3**).

Haemoglobin AA (Hb AA) Normal adult haemoglobin type. Most people have Haemoglobin AA. It is often referred to just as haemoglobin A. (See sections **3.3, 4.2** and **4.3**.)

Haemoglobin C (Hb C) A less common kind of haemoglobin (see sections **4.2, 4.4** and **4.5**).

Haemoglobin electrophoresis A blood test to find out what kind of haemoglobin someone has (see section **8.1**).

Immunised Given an injection to protect against disease (see section **9.1**).

Inherited Passed on to a child by its parents (see section **4**).

Malaria A feverish illness, sometimes fatal, carried by mosquitoes. It occurs mainly in tropical areas (see sections **4, 5, 5.4** and **9.1**).

Painful crisis Pain and sometimes swelling caused when the red blood cells sickle in the blood vessel (see sections **5.5, 5.8** and **5.9**).

Placenta Afterbirth.

Priapism A painful erection of the penis (private parts) caused by sickling in the blood vessels (see section **5.9**).

SC disease (Hb SC) A kind of sickle cell disease. Someone with SC disease has both sickle haemo globin and haemoglobin C in their red blood cells (see sections **4.5** and **6**).

Sequestration When most of the red blood cells collect in the spleen (see section **5.8**).

Sickle With sickle cell disease, the red blood cells sometimes become sickle shaped (see section **3.4**).

Sickle beta-thalassaemia (Hb S Beta-thal) A kind of sickle cell disease. Someone with sickle beta-thalassaemia has genes for sickle haemoglobin and beta-thalassaemia (see sections **4.5** and **7**).

Sickle cell anaemia (Hb SS) A kind of sickle cell disease. Someone with sickle cell anaemia has only sickle haemoglobin in their red blood cells (see sections **4.5** and **5**).

Sickle cell disease The name given to several different kinds of blood disorders in which the red blood cells may sickle (see sections **2, 5, 6** and **7**).

Sickle cell trait (Hb AS) Someone with sickle cell trait has mainly normal haemoglobin but carries the gene for sickle haemoglobin and could pass it on to their children (see section **4.4**).

Sickle haemoglobin (Hb S) A gene for a kind of haemoglobin which sometimes causes the red blood cells to sickle in people with sickle cell disease (see section **3.4**).

Thalassaemia A condition in which the body cannot make enough haemoglobin (see sections **4.4, 4.5** and **7**).

Thalassaemia trait Someone with thalassaemia trait has mainly normal haemoglobin but carries the gene for thalassaemia and could pass it on to their children (see section **4.4**).

Trait A trait is not an illness. Someone with a trait has mainly normal haemoglobin but carries the gene for another kind of haemoglobin and so could pass it on to their children (see section **4.4**).

Transfusion Giving donor blood to someone (see section **9.1**).

Subject Index

References are arranged alphabetically, word by word, taking account of spaces; 'C trait' therefore comes before 'care for sickle cell disease'.

Where there are several references to a topic, any major reference is printed in **bold**; references to the glossary are indicated by 'gl'.